The Homemade Medical Face Mask

Complete Step-By-Step Guide on How to Make Your Own Homemade Medical Face Mask to Protect You From Viruses, Germs, and Bacteria

Paige Elliston

© **Copyright 2020 - All rights reserved.**

The content contained within this book may not be reproduced, duplicated or transmitted without direct written permission from the author or the publisher.

Under no circumstances will any blame or legal responsibility be held against the publisher, or author, for any damages, reparation, or monetary loss due to the information contained within this book, either directly or indirectly.

Legal Notice:

This book is copyright protected. It is only for personal use. You cannot amend, distribute, sell, use, quote or paraphrase any part, or the content within this book, without the consent of the author or publisher.

Disclaimer Notice:

Please note the information contained within this document is for educational and entertainment purposes only. All effort has been executed to present accurate, up to date, reliable, complete information. No warranties of any kind are declared or implied. Readers acknowledge that the author is not engaged in the rendering of legal, financial, medical or professional advice. The content within this book has been derived from various sources. Please consult a licensed professional before attempting any techniques outlined in this book.

By reading this document, the reader agrees that under no circumstances is the author responsible for any losses, direct or indirect, that are incurred as a result of the use of the information contained within this document, including, but not limited to, errors, omissions, or inaccuracies.

Table of Contents

TABLE OF CONTENTS 5

INTRODUCTION 1
- THE MEDICAL MASK: A BRIEF HISTORY 3
  - *Why You Should Make Your Own Masks* 5

CHAPTER 1: WHY MASKS? 9
- HOW DO MASKS WORK? 10
- TYPES OF MASKS 12
  - *How to Wear Masks* 16
  - *Dangers vs Benefits* 21

CHAPTER 2: REUSABLE MASKS 25
- WHY REUSABLE? 26
- MATERIALS TO CONSIDER 27
- DESIGNS AND TECHNIQUES 30
  - *Caring for Your Reusable Mask* 42
  - *Rules of Safety for Reusable Masks* 44

CHAPTER 3: DISPOSABLE MASKS 47
- WHY DISPOSABLE? 48
- MATERIALS TO USE 49
- DESIGNS AND TECHNIQUES 50
  - *Caring for Disposable Masks* 57
  - *Rules of Safety for Disposable Masks* 59

CONCLUSION 61
- NOW YOU KNOW 61
  - *Which Mask Is Right for You?* 63

REFERENCES 67

Introduction

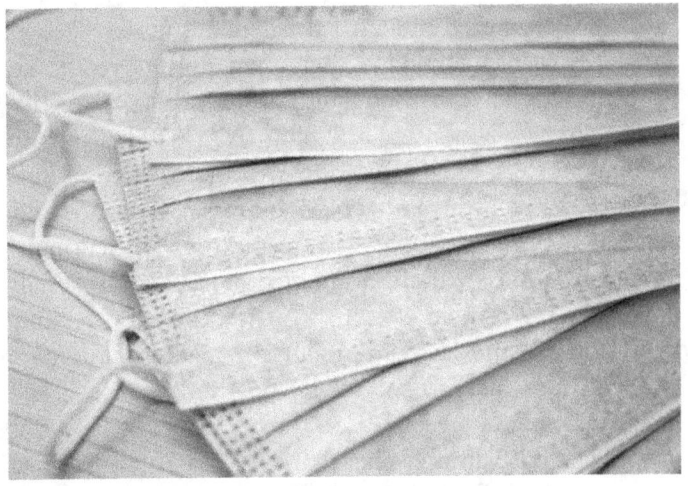

Medical face masks have become a necessity to meet the worldwide threat of airborne contagions and respiratory infections. Though these surgical masks seem easy enough to make at home, there are still many different factors to consider when making and wearing masks of varying designs. Image: Macau Photo Agency on Unsplash.

Medical face masks have become quite an "in-your-face" topic lately. The debate rages on whether it is better to wear masks daily to increase your protection against airborne diseases, viruses, and respiratory infections caused by germs, pollution, and bacteria. It seems that this debate is largely fueled by the global shortage of personal protection equipment (PPE) due to a multitude of respiratory infection outbreaks worldwide. The demand has far outstripped the world's ability to supply medical essentials such as masks and disposable gloves.

This has prompted much of the general public, such as yourself, to begin making their own protective masks. The designs have caused quite a stir on social media, with some designs using anything from padded bras to sanitary towels and coffee filters to improve the safety of these often-ungainly contraptions. Many of the designs are supportive of respiratory functioning; however, some of these homemade masks are woefully inadequate in their design to offer any protection. Additionally, the laymen's focus on making your own medical face mask seems to be on the "patterns" and not on being correctly fitted to the face. This has created a false impression that any mask will protect you. A mask will only offer you protection if it is snugly fitted and if you follow the correct procedures when putting on and removing your mask. We have learned a great deal from history and scientific research about masks, their fit, and protection. Being uninformed about what you choose to wear or not wear as a medical face mask is becoming inexcusable.

The history behind wearing medical face masks is one filled with horrors, misinformation, and propaganda. Today, the wearing of a homemade medical mask may still draw strange looks, yet it is exactly this kind of stereotypical thinking that has cost lives. After all, prevention is better than a cure. You should not wait until you are sick before you start wearing medical face masks. Wear your mask now to prevent getting sick.

This book will equip you with information about which materials are effective to protect you against germs, viruses, and bacterial infections from airborne sources. You will also know what to look for when choosing a design that will offer you maximum protection, while still being comfortable enough to ensure long-term wear.

The Medical Mask: A Brief History

Masks have a rich history of being worn for ceremonial and ritual purposes across the world. However, the first instance of masks being worn for medical purposes was the fearsome masks that doctors wore at the time of the Black Death in Europe during the mid-1300s. This strange mask with glass eye-openings and a beaklike projection, which made the mask look like a dead crow, was designed to keep the smell of putrefaction from the doctors. The "beak" extension was filled with aromatic herbs to cut down on the smell of disease, and the outfit was completed with a long cane to prod the patient with, perhaps serving as the first case of measuring social distancing too.

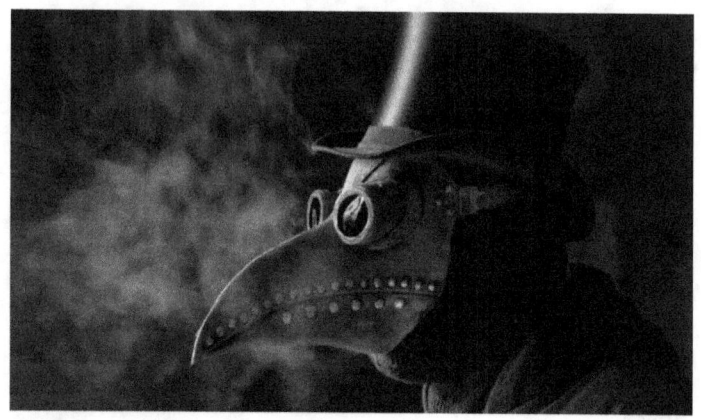

It was a fear-inspiring sight to see a doctor show up with such an outfit, and it may be one of the contributing factors to our modern fear of masks. Image: Kuma Kum on Unsplash.

Many years after the Bubonic Plague ended, the rise of Humanism during the Renaissance of the 14th, 15th, and 16th centuries saw doctors removing their ferocious masks to move into closer proximity to their patients. This led to the modern era of close proximity treatment that we know today.

However, during 1895, a German pathologist discovered that the moisture and particles of human breath could cause open wounds to fester during medical treatment. As a result of this, doctors and nurses began to cover up their mouths with gauze strips as a means to prevent transmission of diseased air onto their patients. These were perhaps the first recorded instances in history of disposable masks for medical purposes. Since then, doctors have routinely worn surgical face masks during medical procedures, invasive therapies, surgeries, and when treating patients in the hospital.

Doctors and nurses are at the frontlines of any respiratory infectious disease crises. Hence, the commercially bought medical face masks and other PPE should be left to supply them. Without doctors and nurses, we would be facing an epic global health care threat. By making your own medical face masks, you would leave the limited stocks of medical-grade PPE for these critical service providers and first responders.

Why You Should Make Your Own Masks

One of the most obvious considerations that may sway you to making your own medical face masks is the increasing cost and increasing shortage of commercially manufactured face masks. Blogger Dave Hamrick (2020) has found that the cost of medical face masks on Amazon.com has increased by a whopping 382% with most stock being sold out faster than new stock can arrive. A tragic side-effect of the scramble for PPE has been the development of a grey market where individuals have bought in bulk and are reselling these items at insane mark-ups. Though governments worldwide have tried to stop this practice from happening, it is still an ongoing struggle.

Additionally, the increasing sale of inferior quality and completely unsanitary products has proliferated on the Internet. A recent viral video of a sweatshop set-up in a third world country showed how children sit on a concrete floor making "sterile" surgical masks by hand. So ordering PPE online may not be a safe bet at all.

Making your own masks will allow you to have a ready supply of masks that are made to a suitable standard to offer you and your family protection. It will also help to reduce the strain on the market of disposable masks that should be reserved for first responders and medical personnel who need to deal with sick people on a daily basis.

A benefit of making your own masks, apart from the obvious fashion statement that you could make, is that you can tailor it to be an exact and more comfortable fit. High-quality masks such as the N95 masks are far from comfortable and are known for bruising the face with prolonged wear.

Relying on a constant supply of disposable masks also creates a problem of how to dispose of these masks once they have been worn. Disposable masks, gloves, and other PPE are considered medical waste, and these should be incinerated at a medical facility. Disposing of them in your trash at home poses a serious health risk. With the global increase in this form of medical waste, it creates a serious threat of pollution. Most surgical-type masks are made from materials that are also not biodegradable. This means that if we dispose of these masks in an unwise manner, the problems will be there for many years to come. Another concern is that these contaminated masks could start polluting the world's freshwater supply. This should be a real concern as viruses and bacteria can spread through contact, water, and the air. Being responsible means safeguarding our global futures.

Given the cost of disposable masks, the temptation to wear them several times over also becomes greater, and this defeats the whole purpose—which is to keep you protected. There are some online sources claiming that disposable masks can be re-sterilized by washing, though the research on this is still inconclusive. However, washing these masks at home may further expose your home and family to any contaminants, viruses, and bacteria that you may have inadvertently trapped in your disposable masks. It is not a simple matter of chucking these masks in the wash with the rest of your laundry.

This is where the proper care for your masks is essential. Homemade medical masks are more resilient to the processes of cleaning them, and with an effective and hygienic strategy in place, you can easily clean them and be assured of their safe and continued protection.

So grab your sewing kit, some enthusiasm, and a pinch of creativity. Time to mask up!

Chapter 1:

Why Masks?

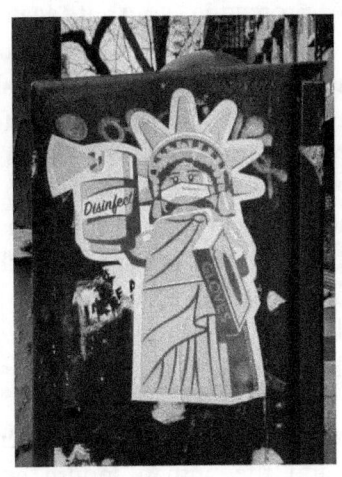

The human body has several contact points with the outside environment, the skin being the largest. However, the mouth, nose, and eyes are the most vulnerable to absorbing foreign materials such as dust, bacteria, viruses, sputum, and other undesirable particles. Covering the mouth and nose with a mask is a safe way to minimize your risk of contracting any airborne diseases. Image: John Tyson on Unsplash.

How Do Masks Work?

Medical face masks work on the principle of forming a semi-impermeable barrier to stop foreign matter from entering the nose and mouth during the inhalation process. This barrier is only semi-impermeable as you still need to breathe. The choice of mask will depend on what you are protecting yourself against. Different contaminants come in different-sized particles, hence, the need for a denser mask or even a mask with a filter when you are in a high-risk area for biological contaminants that may come in smaller particle sizes.

A medical face mask is a covering that completely covers the mouth and nose, separating the respiratory tract from the surrounding environment. It can be attached by elastic bands or surgical ties. Some masks have filters, while others do not.

Masks need to make a tight-sealing barrier between the mask's edges and the human mouth and nose area. Only then will the mask offer effective protection. Additionally, masks that are being removed and replaced frequently and often incorrectly increase the risk of contamination through foreign particles that have collected at the edges of the masks.

Masks do limit the amount of oxygen that you can easily obtain through breathing. Hence, masks are not recommended to be worn during strenuous exercise. Placing the body's natural breathing mechanism under strain by cutting off air supply would not only be uncomfortable but also counterproductive. Since the body requires more oxygen during physical activities, it might explain why the recent spate of respiratory diseases have hit health and fitness facilities like gyms the hardest. A body that can breathe effectively is a body that is healthy. Since our skin is quite capable of repelling most airborne assaults from diseases, it is through our mouths and noses that we become exposed to particles that cause illness.

Wearing masks is also not only about preventing yourself from contracting an airborne disease. It is also about not sharing an airborne disease that you may have such as the common flu. In this sense, the mask will stop your coughs, sneezes, and even your breath from releasing droplets of moisture that contain harmful biological matter that could infect others who breathe in this contaminated air.

Coughing can spread contaminated air as far as six meters, while sneezing can spread it as far as eight meters from the person who coughed or sneezed. These droplets also have a variable "hang-time" that is dependent on the size of the sneeze particles, airflow, and even heat. Most of us are able to cover our mouths when we cough, though a sneeze can surprise us and escape before we can react. A medical face mask is very helpful in these instances as it protects you from other people's coughing and sneezing as well as protecting other people from yours.

A secondary consideration is that when we cough into our hands, we are simply transferring these contagions to our hands to be further spread by physical contact. A mask would help to catch any biological matter released from our respiratory tract to protect those around us.

In recent days, the Center for Disease Control (CDC) and the World Health Organization (WHO) have both begun to recommend the wearing of medical face masks when out in public as a preventive measure against airborne contaminants. Masks offer the protection of limiting your exposure to airborne particles from sneezes and coughing. Additionally, they also serve as a reminder for you not to touch your face with your hands. This is important since the hands carry residue from every surface that they may have come into contact with. The hands become taxis for the microbes and other harmful particles that can cause respiratory diseases and conditions such as sinusitis. Hence, the need to frequently wash your hands with soap.

Types of Masks

Masks can be split into different categories based on their ability to shield the mask wearer from different-sized particles, as well as whether these masks are for single-use (being disposable masks) or are reusable (after being sanitized).

Choosing a mask is not simply about wrapping a piece of material around your face. There are many different masks, mask designs, and mask materials to consider when choosing a mask. For the sake of clarity, we will consider the two main classifications of medical face masks, namely the medical or surgical face mask and the respirator-type face mask that is known for a reinforced dome that covers the mouth and nose.

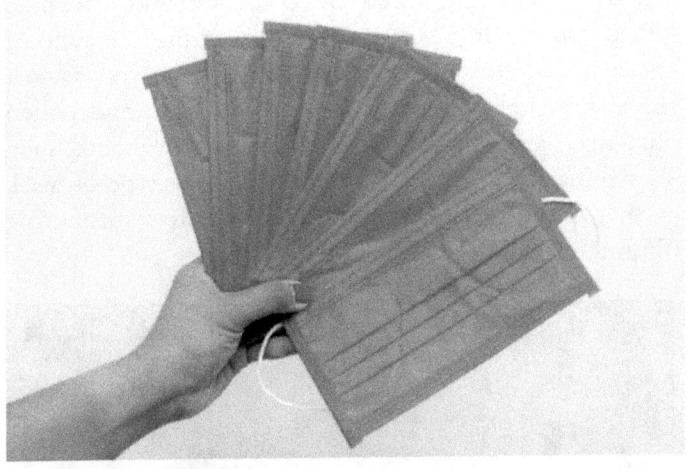

The surgical type of face mask is a simplistic design that allows for mass production. It covers the most direct forms of airflow both into and out of the mouth and nose. However, it is often not correctly fitted to the individual wearer and can become compromised. Image: Macau Photo Agency on Unsplash.

The most common design is the surgical face mask that we know from popular medical dramas on TV. These masks are lightweight and used to be cheap to purchase. As a moderately effective means of controlling coughing and sneezing, these masks have also become popular in the catering industry with many workers who are involved with and handle food being required to wear these masks.

The pleated design allows for the mask to expand to better cover the nose and mouth, extending down under the chin. Simple elastic bands tie the mask onto the ears. This type of mask is effective in containing larger droplets produced by coughing and sneezing. Once you become accustomed to wearing this type of mask, it is also quite handy for protecting you against environmental pollutants such as dust, gas, and pollen that may be responsible for respiratory problems such as asthma and sinusitis. The benefit of this type of mask is that it is more comfortable than the respirators that fit much more tightly.

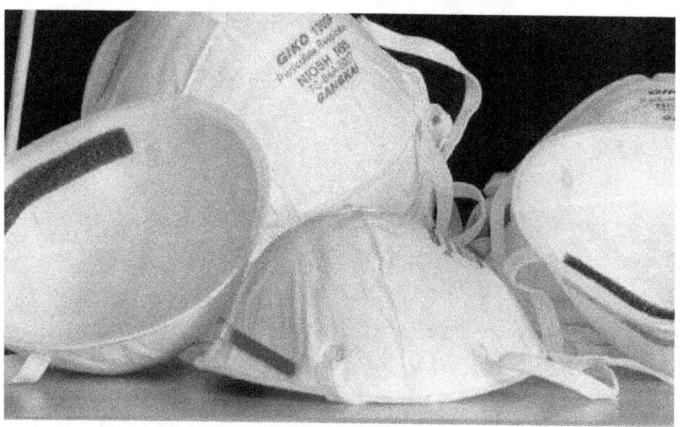

The N95 medical mask is a rigid structure that encapsulates the nose and mouth area offering protection from 95% of all foreign particles. Image (cropped): C Drying on Unsplash.

The much sturdier and tighter fitting N95-type mask is considered to be the best form of PPE (not including a hazmat suit), and it is tested to prevent 95% of all airborne particles, viruses, bacteria, and other disease RNA from reaching the airways. For someone who is already sick, this mask is also the best protection that they can offer those around them.

This mask is also known as a respirator since it keeps the air from circulating away from the nose and mouth, forming a contained environment. Air is only available through the filtration process that the mask facilitates. Due to this very specific functioning of cutting off all free-flowing airflow, the N95 respirator fits really tightly around the nose and mouth. It is known for cutting off circulation and causing facial bruising.

As such, the N95 is by far the least comfortable of PPE masks available to the general public. To ensure a snug fit, the N95 respirator comes with a metal strip to conform the nose area to your own nose, cutting off any escape of air along the sides of your nose. It also has tight-fitting double elastic bands that are cut to ensure the mask fits exactly with its shaped form along the contours of your face.

This type of medical face mask, or respirator, is not recommended for extended wear. Given the price and its apparently resilient construction, the temptation to re-wear the mask more than once is also greater, making these masks a health hazard.

How to Wear Masks

Wearing masks may not be as easy or as simple as it seems. In a world where we are becoming more accustomed to seeing people out in public wearing an assortment of masks, it has become almost comical to see the different (and usually incorrect) ways in which people wear medical face masks and respirators. Medical professionals advise a specific method of putting on and removing your medical face mask. This method may seem excessive, but without following proper protocol, medical face masks can become a danger to you and to others.

Follow these steps when putting on a medical face mask or a respirator:

- **Wash Your Hands**

Your hands will, in all likelihood, touch all the different parts of the mask as you are busy fitting it. Make sure that you have washed your hands for at least 20 seconds using warm water and disinfectant soap. Don't simply rub your hands together. You need to clean the palms, fingers, nails, nail beds, and the sides of the thumbs as well as the sides of your hands.

Be cautious of loose jewelry such as bracelets and rings that may hoard contaminants only to deposit these on the inside of your mask.

- **Tuck Your Hair**

With a medical face mask being designed to fit snugly and to minimize the number of times that you touch your face, you would also be well-served to tuck your hair away from your face. If you have long hair, tie it back while you are fitting your mask but **before** washing your hands. Human hair can also contain contaminants.

For men, the issue of the beard has been a historical one, and the evidence is still inconclusive in this regard. Some medical professionals believe that a beard interferes with the correct fit of a medical face mask. Facial whiskers may indeed push the face mask away from the optimal placement, allowing contaminated air to reach the mouth and nose.

Should you already be sick, the hairs on your face could provide additional surface area for germs to hide away in. However, practicing good personal hygiene and washing your beard regularly will go a long way toward ensuring your (and everyone else's) health.

- **Apply the Mask**

When picking up the new medical mask to put it on your face, you need to only take it by the elastics or by the straps. Do not touch the inside of the mask at all. Slip the elastics over your ears one at a time, positioning it comfortably. If the mask has straps, you need to tie these effectively, but ensure that you can untie them later when you need to remove the mask too. With the surgical mask type, you need to gently separate the folds to open the mask out to cover the bottom of your chin and reach up to the bridge of your nose.

With the respirator-type mask, you need to take hold of both elastics in one hand, while supporting the body of the mask with the other. Take care to only touch the outside of the mask. Slip both elastics over your head at the same time. Settle the body of the mask into place, then spread out the elastics to be more comfortable. It is recommended that the elastics should cross at the back of your head to ensure a tight seal is achieved and even pressure of the mask on your face.

- **Shape the Mask**

Commercially bought masks come with either a metal wire (in surgical masks) or metal plate (in respirators) on the nose part to allow for the effective shaping of the mask. You should press on the sides of your nose to create a shape that matches the lines of your nose. There should be no gaps between the mask and your nose or the area under your eyes.

Creating a tight fit is possible due to these metal shapers that you find at the top of these masks. It is essential to stop air from escaping from next to the nose and under the eyes. A correct fit will also stop your glasses from fogging up.

The next time that you touch your mask should only be when you are ready to remove and dispose of your mask. Don't fiddle with it as this increases the risk of contamination.

Follow these steps to remove your medical face mask:

- **Think Disposal**

Before you remove your used medical face mask or respirator, you need to plan on and be prepared to dispose of it. If it is a reusable mask, you need to be ready to store it safely until you can take steps to sterilize it. Don't take your mask off and only then start thinking of what to do with it. Be prepared—this will limit the chances of you spreading a contagion.

Have a plastic bag (preferably a Ziplock bag) that you can store the used mask in to either dispose of at home by burning or for sanitizing at home. It is probably a good idea to label the packet so that there is no confusion that it contains a **used** medical face mask. Open the bag so that you can easily insert the used mask once you have removed it. Remember, a used medical face mask is hazardous and biological waste. It is not a candy wrapper.

- **Remove the Mask**

When you are ready with your storage bag, you can begin removing the mask. If it is tied over your ears with elastics, then slip off both ear loops to lower the mask horizontally away from the face. Do not shake the mask as this may disperse particles contained in the mask. Do not touch the body of the mask; instead, slip it into the plastic packet. Seal the packet.

- **Wash Your Hands**

With the used mask secured in the packet, you can now wash your hands. Again, do so for at least 20 seconds, making sure to wash every nook and cranny of your hands, nails, and fingers. Air drying your hands is best, but a paper towel can also be used. If you have a spray-on disinfectant handy, you may want to spray the outside of your plastic packet.

- **Wash or Wipe Your Face**

It may seem extreme, but a good preventive step is to wash your face with warm, soapy water or to wipe your face with a disinfectant wipe. While you were removing your mask, you may have inadvertently dislodged particles from the mask. These may have landed on your face, so it's a good idea to clean up your face too.

As a last precaution, place your plastic packet with the used mask somewhere safe where uninformed persons will not accidentally open the packet. If you are able to throw the mask and its packet away, then do so in a covered bin. Should you intend to sterilize the mask for reuse, you may need to place it where you can control who has access to it until you have sanitized the mask.

A final note on mask placement. Masks are uncomfortable, especially if you have not been previously wearing them. It is your choice to wear a mask or not. If you wear one, then you should wear it correctly, or else it may do more harm than good. You should keep it in place until you remove it. Do not lower the mask to "catch a breather" or to take a smoke break or to have a cup of tea, and then pull it back into place. Once you have "broken" the air seal of the mask with your face, you have opened up the possibilities for contamination. Using a mask to only cover the mouth and leaving your nose open to "help you breathe" will only expose you to more contaminants. A medical face mask should be worn correctly or not at all.

Dangers vs Benefits

On the whole, prevention is always better than cure. The logic then holds that wearing a protective medical face mask is better than not wearing one. Preventing respiratory infections by wearing a medical face mask is also a much more cost-effective option, especially when you are wearing a reusable face mask. This seems like the best option then.

However, there are also downsides to wearing medical face masks.

- **False Sense of Security**

Wearing a medical face mask may give the wearer a false sense of security. It could make people believe they are more protected than they actually are. This could result in people not avoiding crowds or not observing good social distancing practices. Our instinct is to avoid people who we can see are sick. Yet with a mask on, you may be tempted to spend time in close proximity around sick people when you should keep a safe distance.

- **Incorrect Fit**

When you do not fit your medical face mask correctly, you risk exposing yourself to even more contaminants and airborne diseases. People are sometimes ignorant of this and may end up only covering their mouths, leaving their nasal openings uncovered. Incorrect fit may expose the wearer to even more contaminated surfaces.

- **Reuse**

Given that masks have become much more costly, and they can also be harder to find, people are likely to wear masks longer than they should. A soggy mask is a danger as it absorbs sputum particles and increases your risk of exposure. People are also likely to reuse masks that they think are not "used" enough to try and save money. This could become a serious hazard when a family shares masks or if you are unsure whether someone has touched your mask or not.

- **Increased Hygiene Neglect**

Wearing a mask may also lead to people forgetting to follow other personal hygiene protocols such as washing hands and maintaining a degree of interpersonal separation or social distancing. When you forget to wash your hands or wash them less frequently, you are increasing the risk that your hands may spread germs from other surfaces to parts of your body such as your face, neck, and arms. Medical face masks are only effective when they are fitted by clean hands and when you wash your hands after removing the mask.

- **Increased Medical Waste**

The reality is that when you wear disposable medical face masks or disposable surgical gloves, you are creating hazardous waste. This waste has to go somewhere. It needs to be treated responsibly; otherwise, you will simply be spreading germs. This can make medical face masks and surgical gloves a danger to society.

- **Worsen Respiratory Conditions**

Though medical face masks can improve your chances of avoiding the contraction of respiratory diseases, they can increase the difficulty with which you breathe. People suffering from asthma, sinusitis, and other breathing conditions may struggle to get sufficient air supply when wearing a medical face mask or respirator. The feeling of being covered may lead to anxiety and feelings of suffocation, worsening breathing conditions.

Wearing a medical face mask is a choice. As such, it also comes with a responsibility to act with awareness, care for others, and have full knowledge of mask usage. Wearing a face mask or a respirator is not a right. It is a decision that you make, and you should be held accountable for how that choice impacts others. Wearing a medical face mask can certainly offer increased protection to you and your family from respiratory diseases, but this is only the case when you wear these PPE correctly, dispose of them responsibly, and maintain these masks before and after use.

Chapter 2:

Reusable Masks

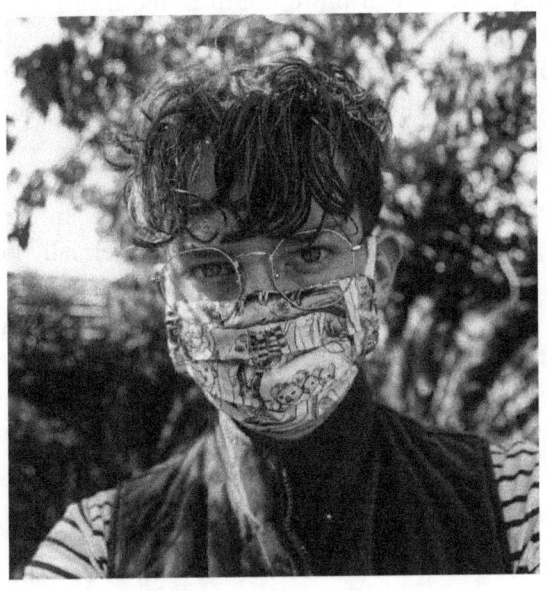

Making your own medical face masks can be fun, and with some creativity, they can become a fashion statement and a functional PPE. Image: Gryffyn M on Unsplash.

Why Reusable?

The obvious reasons to make and wear your own reusable medical face masks are probably the increasing cost and limited availability of disposable medical face masks and respirators. However, making your own medical face masks can also mean that you can create a functional yet much more comfortable face mask. Our bodies are not all the same dimensions, and where one person may be comfortable with a five-centimeter elastic band behind their ears, someone else may need double that length.

Comfort is the main reason why people fiddle with their medical face masks, whether commercially bought or homemade. When you keep readjusting the mask because it is uncomfortable, you are defeating the whole point of the mask. The mask should fit correctly, comfortably, and remain in place until it is removed. Unlike a hat that you can put on or take off as you like, a medical face mask should be seen as a "fixture."

Wearing a medical face mask in public or for prolonged periods of time, such as during the school day, may also not be everyone's cup of tea. Certainly, your children may not be wild about the concept. Creating a fun, funky, and functional medical face mask is a great way to ensure that your children will continue to wear their medical face masks while you are not looking.

When a medical face mask becomes part of your wardrobe, you are also more likely to wear it on a daily basis, and you will also make sure not to lose it when out in public. No matter which way you look at a reusable medical face mask, it is a very useful addition to your life.

Materials to Consider

When choosing a material to use in making your own reusable face masks, you need to keep in mind which materials are suitable for protecting against different-sized particles that may penetrate your mask. Most environmental factors such as spores, dust, and pollen are sized up to one micron. Bacteria and spores are also larger-sized molecules. These larger molecules can be caught by thinner materials that may prevent protection against infections.

Robertson (2020) reported on research by Smart Air into different household materials and their efficacy in offering protection as homemade face masks. The research found some interesting results.

For large-sized (one micron) molecules such as bacteria, dust, and contaminants such as gasses, the star performers were:

- **Dish Towels**

The common kitchen dish towel or terry cloth surprised everyone by successfully stopping 83% of large airborne particles. As an added bonus, it is a hard-wearing material that can be bleached, washed, and even heated to sterilize the masks made of this material for reuse. When folded, this material's protection factor increased, though this made the mask heavy and complicated breathing through the mask.

- **Cotton-Blend T-Shirt**

Next on the list was the cotton-blend T-shirt. It managed to successfully trap 74% of the larger particles. Again, with multiple layers, this protection factor increased. This is a flexible and easy-wearing material that can face up to rigorous washing and bleaching if needed. As a bonus, you can paint on this material, creating your own fashion statement.

- **Pillowcases**

A pillowcase managed to stop 62% of the larger microbes, while an antimicrobial pillowcase stopped 65% of larger molecules. This material is also easily found, very friendly to sewing, and can be washed, sterilized, and heated to destroy biological matter trapped in it after the mask has been used. Masks of this material wear comfortably, and you could easily add a filter to increase its protection factor. It's also paint-friendly, so you can get your kids involved.

For smaller particles (0.1 microns and smaller) such as viruses, the same materials also performed well, ranking only slightly lower than the commercially bought surgical masks. The dish towel stopped 73% of particles, the cotton-blend T-shirt stopped 70%, while the pillowcases stopped 57% of these smaller particles. This means that wearing a homemade medical face mask increased the wearer's protection by at least 50% against viruses. Double layering these materials added at least 2% protection to the above materials. This leaves some room for innovation in designing your own homemade medical face masks.

When considering the materials to add to your mask as an additional filter, the best by far is a high-efficiency particulate air (HEPA) vacuum bag. This material is not very flexible, but when added as a layer over the nose and mouth area of the mask, it increases the protection to 95% for larger particles and 86% for smaller particles. Coffee filters are also proving a popular choice as filter material due to their tight weave and ability to retain small particles quite well.

Now that you know what to use, it's time to look at different designs and choose a method and style that works for you.

Designs and Techniques

Now that you have decided on which materials are best for your individual protection needs, it is time to start making the mask. Firstly, disinfect your hands, all surfaces, and any tools that you may be using. This is important, as you want to keep the masks that you make as clean and infection-free as possible. Wiping surfaces with rubbing alcohol is probably best, though you can also clean with warm water and soap.

Basic Surgical Mask Design

This is one of the easiest designs to make, and you only need to have minimal sewing skills to make this mask successfully. Williams (2020) has provided a good basic design.

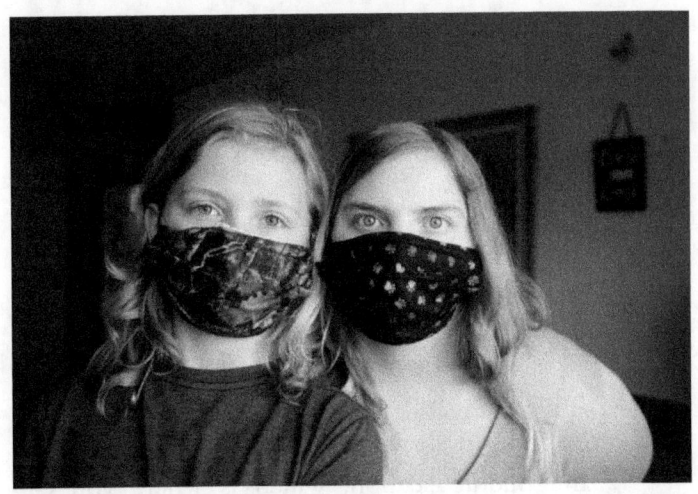

This mask can be customized by adding a second layer to improve the mask's protection. This second layer can be painted or made of different patterned materials. Be careful to pinch the nose section's wire to conform to the shape of your nose to improve the fit. Image: Sharon McCutcheon on Unsplash.

What you'll need:

- 15 x 8-inch tightly woven material such as pillowcases or T-shirt fabric
- Two 7-inch elastics or two hair ties
- One 2-inch pipe cleaner or medium-thickness galvanized wire
- Pins and cotton
- Scissors, measuring tape, and sewing machine

How to make it:

1. Sew a half-inch seam along the 15-inch sides of the material.
2. Insert the pipe cleaner or wire into the top seam, centering it, and securing it in place with a vertical stitch.
3. Pin elastics to the short sides, fold the fabric over, and sew.
4. Turning the mask so that it is right-side down on your work surface, fold in a one-inch pleat from the top and also from the bottom, stitching it down from both sides, except for the middle section, which is where you can insert a filter piece of about 4 x 2 inches.
5. Fold three more pleats, stitching these along the edges of the mask only. This will give your mask the folded appearance of commercial masks and also give you flexibility and allow the mask to expand to fit your face.

And you're done.

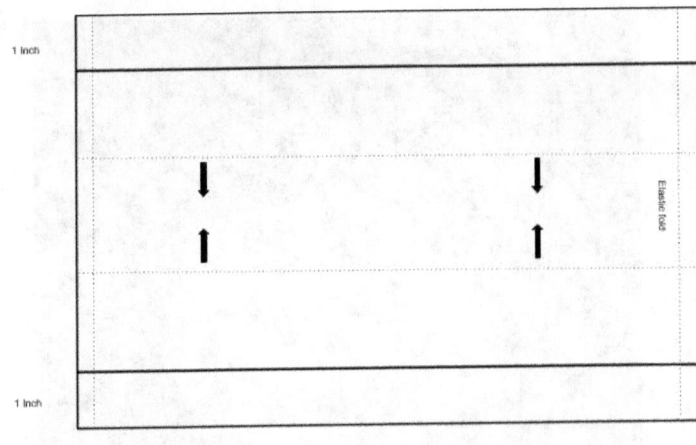

For a more exact template of the pleats and folds, you might follow this template. Template one.

Shaped Mask Design

This mask is shaped to give more protection along the nose area. You could also shape it downwards to improve the fit over your chin. Again, remember to sanitize all work surfaces, tools, and materials where possible.

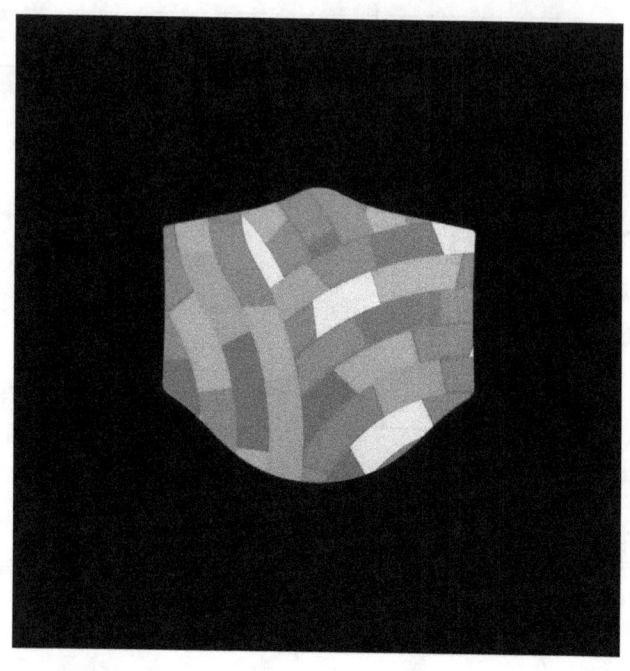

The basic design when shaped both at the top and bottom may look like this. Image: Visuals on Unsplash.

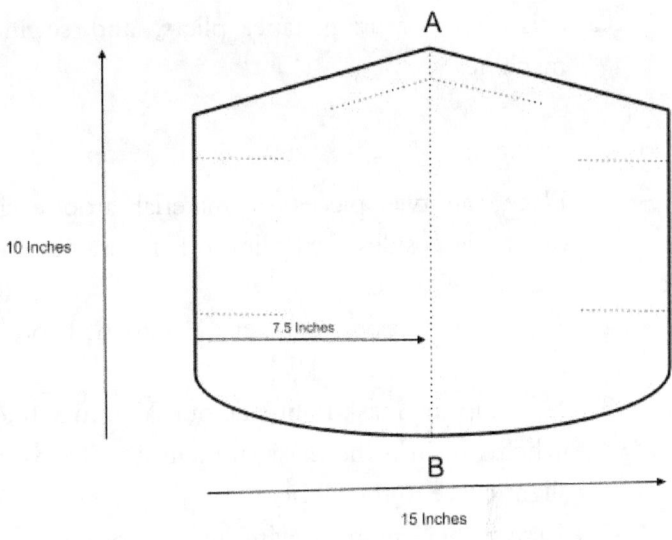

The template of the mask can be cut according to these lines. Template two.

What you'll need:

- ❏ Two mask cut-outs according to the provided template
- ❏ Two 7-inch elastics or two hair ties. Alternatively, you could add four seamed straps that you could tie behind your head. These would need to be about 15 inches each.
- ❏ One 2-inch pipe cleaner or medium-thickness galvanized wire (you could also use a paper clip folded open or thick-quality aluminum foil).
- ❏ Pins and cotton

- ❏ Scissors, measuring tape, pliers, and sewing machine

How to make it:

1. Place the two pieces of material atop each other, right sides facing inward. Insert pins to secure the fabric.
2. Sew the long sides together (A onto A, B onto B).
3. Now flip the mask right-side out. You may find it helps to iron the mask, though it will have a slight curve to the fabric.
4. Taking the length of wire, use pliers to make small loops at both ends. This will make sure that the wire doesn't poke you in the face when you are wearing the mask. Insert the wire into the mask, centering it in place at the top of curve A. Secure it with pins and sew along it as indicated on the template. Finish this off by sewing in a few vertical stitches to secure the wire and prevent it from slipping out.
5. Now, fold the sides inward. You may insert the elastic already, sewing it into the seam as you go, or you could sew the edges, leaving a small opening at the corners so that you could later thread the elastic through.
6. You can decide whether you want to make ear loops with the elastic or if you would like to

make one continuous elastic band that forms two larger loops that you can use to make a set of double elastics to fit over your head (like the N95 mask's fittings).
7. If you have opted for the straps, then sew the edged straps onto the corners of the mask. For comfort, you may want to sew the top straps at a slight angle so that the straps will go straight upward toward your ears when you wear it, limiting unnecessary folds and bulges.
8. Optional: You can also add small tucks sewn onto the sides of the mask as per the template. By sewing the center line as per the template, you will also be able to reinforce the area over your nose and mouth. This is to improve the fit.

For an even more padded fit, you could use the padded cups for bras, if your local clothing retail store is open, or you could use your bra cups as is, simply cutting off any excess material that sticks out beyond the template above. You would insert the bra cup in between the two layers of fabric before step 1 above.

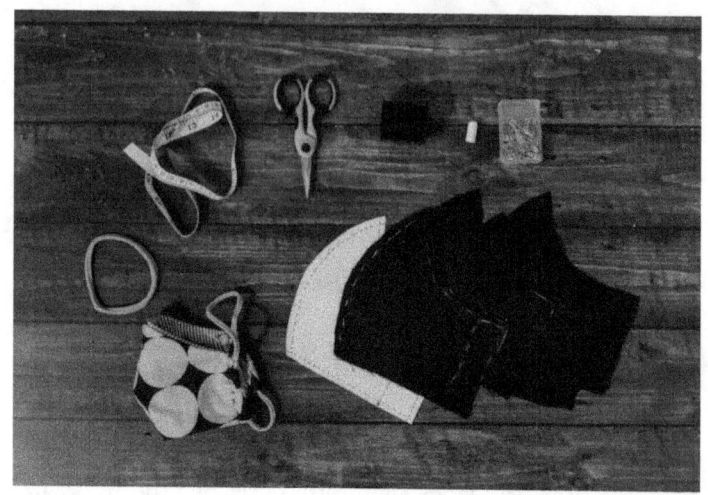

Making your own reusable medical face masks is not as difficult as you would imagine. It will allow you to take control of your own health and protect yourself and your family, and it can become a fun activity for the whole family. Image: Kelly Sikkema on Unsplash.

Duckbill Face Mask

This mask is ideal for people who are sensitive to having material pressing on their faces. It is also ideal for men with beards since the mask's shape is formed to leave enough breathing room.

If you struggle with moisture from your breath, you can add an additional lining to the mask to absorb unnecessary moisture. For this purpose, you can use folded kitchen paper towels or even a maxi pad.

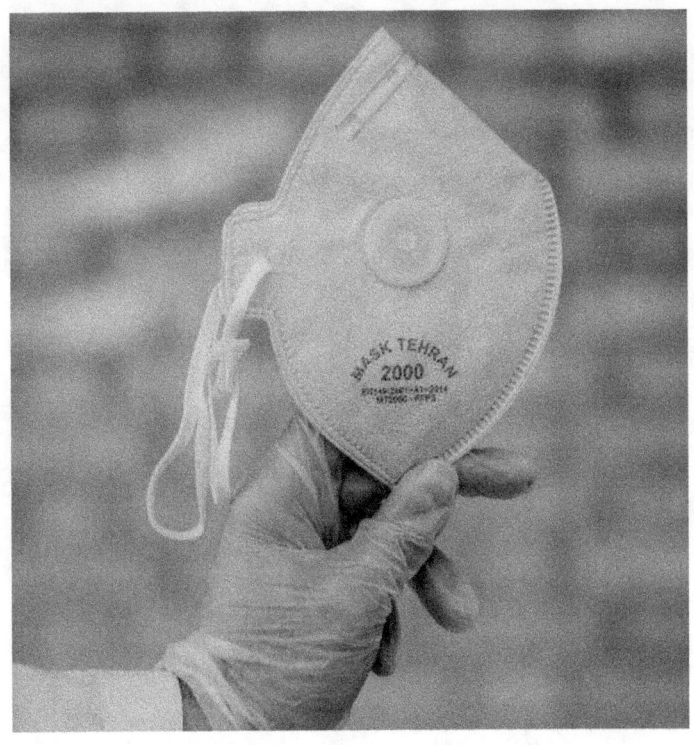

The duckbill mask design is one of the more unconventional mask patterns that also enjoys commercial use. The "bill" can be flattened either vertically (as in the picture) or horizontally. Image: Askan Forouzani on Unsplash.

What you will need:

- ❏ Two cut-outs as per template of polycotton or sheeting
- ❏ One cut-out as per template of batting

- ❏ 35 inches of bias binding or 2-inch wide cotton ribbon
- ❏ 12-inch length of elastic
- ❏ 3-inch length of metal wire or double-folded strip of aluminum foil
- ❏ Scissors and needle
- ❏ Cotton and sewing pins
- ❏ Sewing machine

How to make it:

1. Cut out the template of the duckbill mask, twice in your chosen fabric and once in the batting.
2. Layer these cut-outs with the batting sandwiched between the two layers of fabric (make sure to have the fabric sides facing right-side-out).
3. Fold part A onto part B with the fabric you want on the outside of your mask on the inside of the fold. Pin this in place and sew along the diagonal edges.
4. Push the sewn "cup shape" outward so that the mask is now facing the right-side out. Iron to flatten any creases.
5. Using the bias binding or cotton ribbon, neatly edge the outer lines of the mask (15 x 15-inch sides). You now have the typical duckbill shape.

6. Using a little extra bias binding or cotton ribbon, attach the wire section as shown on the template to create a nose mold on the upper edge of the mask. You could also attach the wire by bending it into a V-shape over the edge of the duckbill shape (both options are shown on the template). Remember to bend the ends of the wire into small loops to make it more comfortable to wear. Pliers can be used to bend the wire or you can use your hands.
7. Next place the mask into position on your face, attach the elastic to one side (depending on whether the duckbill is horizontal or vertical), and measure the length of elastic required for your head to create a comfortable but securely fitting mask. Now sew both ends of the elastic into place.

And you are ready to quack away into a healthy day. If you find that the mask gets moist from your breath, you can add a padded layer of paper towel to help absorb the moisture on the inside. However, if you need to replace the towel, you should also change to a fresh mask.

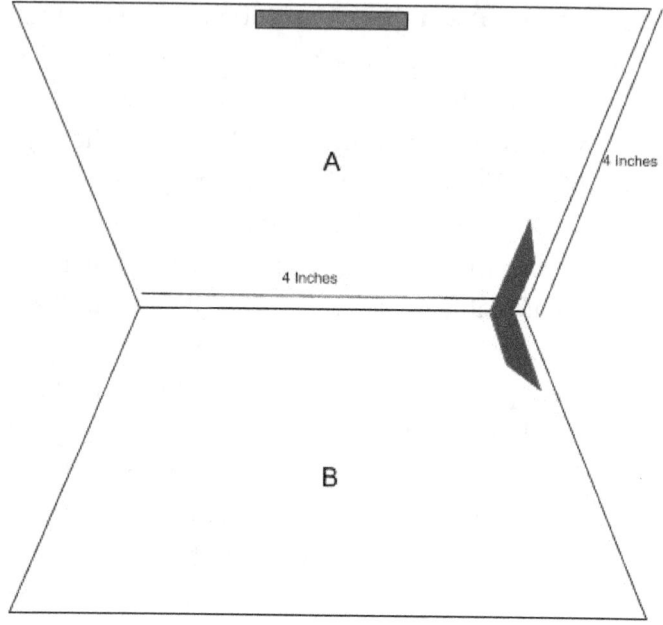

Template Three: Duckbill Mask.

Caring for Your Reusable Mask

A reusable mask is designed for comfort and for its ability to be sanitized so that you can use it again. It does not mean that you can wear it over and over again without sanitizing it. The same protocols you apply to disposable masks should be used here. If you have to take off the mask, you should put on a fresh one, securing the used mask in a plastic packet until you are able to wash or sanitize the mask.

When making your mask, it is advisable to use two different color fabrics. This will help you remember what side is the outside, and you should always keep the same side facing outward for added hygiene.

To sanitize your mask, you should wash it in warm water with sufficient amounts of soap to produce a good lather and foam. Scrub the mask vigorously. You might consider using a nail brush or an old toothbrush to scrub at the seams. The goal is to remove as much of any possible contaminant as possible. To dry the mask, hang it in a well-ventilated area, preferably in direct sunlight. Most germs do not enjoy the UV radiation of direct sunlight.

If you are living in an area where you can't hang your masks in direct sunlight to dry, you might consider tumble drying the mask as this will add the element of heat exposure, which most germs are also sensitive to. Most tumble driers can reach temperatures of 80° Celsius or 175° Fahrenheit, which is quite sufficient to kill off any lurking germs.

Additionally, you may consider adding bleach, peroxide, or alcohol to the wash if you feel that your mask may have been exposed to serious contamination such as when visiting with a sick person.

Fabrics such as T-shirts and pillowcases are quite resilient and will hold up well to bleaching, scrubbing, heat, and sunlight. However, the elastics are likely to take a beating, and you may need to replace these more frequently. You might consider this when deciding on a design for your mask. To allow for you to change the elastics regularly, you may opt for punching a small hole and edging this with an eyelet or grommet. This would let you change the elastics on a regular basis without having to undo any of your sewing.

You should, however, remember to clean vigorously around any additional elements such as eyelets, buttons, or Velcro since these are likely to attract more contaminants. This is also why you should refrain from "decorating" the mask with fancy trimmings, beads, or ribbons as these will result in you not cleaning your mask as effectively.

Rules of Safety for Reusable Masks

Reusable medical face masks should meet strict requirements in their fit, care, and the personal hygiene routines that you combine with them. They do not substitute safe practices such as washing your hands regularly, avoiding touching your face, and gargling water in your throat to avoid infections. Here are some rules to take cognizance of:

1. Wash your hands before putting on your mask, as well as before and after you take your mask off.
2. Store used masks in a plastic packet until they can be cleaned.
3. Store new masks in a closed container to avoid contamination before you wear them.

4. Check that the mask fits snugly, and there should be no openings where you can feel air being "sucked in" as you breathe normally.
5. Make sure that the elastics have sufficient tension in them to pull the mask snuggly onto your face. Change tired or worn-out elastics regularly. A medical face mask should not sag downward from your face.
6. Check the fabric regularly to ensure that the material hasn't split or worn through. Especially focus on the nose area as the wire nose piece is prone to rust and could damage the fabric easily.
7. Never wear a fabric or reusable face mask more than once. If you need to take it off for lunchtime, then take this opportunity to replace it with a fresh mask, bagging the used one to be cleaned later.

Reusable medical face masks are a sensible solution to our modern era where we face pollution, disease, and other contaminants that may influence the quality of the air that we breathe or make us fall sick. Having a mask available that you can trust will help you face the world with increased confidence. Going reusable helps to cut down on pollution, and it also helps by leaving in stock disposable masks for healthcare workers who need these on an ongoing daily basis. But what about when you can't use a reusable mask? You can also make your own disposable masks.

Chapter 3:

Disposable Masks

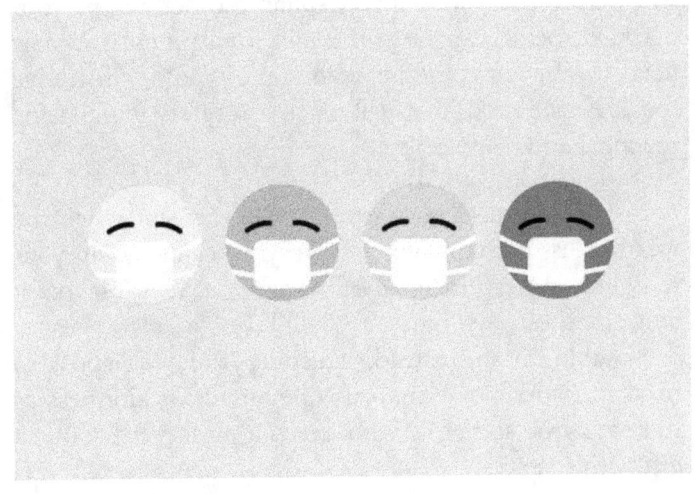

A disposable mask is a face mask that is designed to be worn only once. It may be nearly as efficient at protecting the wearer as any expensive and tested commercial medical face mask. The secret lies in the correct fit and in using suitable materials to make a temporary or disposable face mask. Image: Visuals on Unsplash.

Why Disposable?

There are many reasons why you may need to wear a disposable mask. You might be away and may not be able to safely pack and keep your reusable mask to take it home with you for cleaning. You might have had an accident that compromised your reusable mask, such as snapped elastics, accidentally spilling something on your mask, or being caught in the rain. In a pinch, you may need to quickly come up with some type of protective medical face mask that will offer you safety while being practical and disposable.

A disposable mask may offer you a way out when the weather is perhaps rainy, and you can't wash your reusable masks. Instead of wearing a reusable mask twice without washing, it would be safer to wear a disposable mask instead. Keeping a few disposable masks in your purse may also be an act of kindness as there may be someone who needs a mask who you can gift with one.

If you are not the sewing type, then a disposable mask may be a great way to protect yourself on the odd occasion that you have to nip into the corner market to buy a loaf of bread. Making a disposable mask can be a very quick process, taking as little as five minutes, and best of all, it's really easy.

Materials to Use

When considering materials that may be used for disposable masks, you should keep in mind that they should be disposable and not made out of materials that will not degrade. Otherwise, they could end up spreading diseases during the disposal process and when in landfills.

Materials can be sorted under porous materials such as papers and tissues and non-porous materials such as vinyl, plastics, metal, etc. The porous materials will be more flexible and tend to allow you to breathe easier, while the non-porous materials will be less flexible but could offer better protection against foreign particles in the air. If you choose to use a filter in your design, remember to place a second layer between the filter and your mouth to prevent breathing in any harmful materials such as fibers that may be shed by the filter materials.

Disposable masks may also be made using fabrics such as handkerchiefs, scarves, and bandanas if this is all that you have available. In this case, the term disposable is meant to indicate that you will probably be throwing the mask away once it has been worn since you have not sewn the mask, and it can't be washed then.

No matter the material that you choose, you need to remember to keep it as hygienic as possible before and during the manufacturing process as well as when you put your disposable mask on.

A note of caution: When using glues and other fasteners, remember that these will be in close contact with your face and should not have a chemical smell that might lead to drowsiness. When using paper and cardboard, be careful of sharp edges that may cut or scratch your face.

Paper, plastics, and other disposable materials have not been substantively tested in their ability to repel foreign particles or protect from infections; however, given the density of paper, it can realistically be expected to offer at least a 60% safety rate.

In the end, the material that you choose will only be as efficient as the design of your mask. The real benefit of disposable homemade face masks is that they are cheaply and quickly made. This makes them ideal for people who can't (or won't) sew and for bachelors (and bachelorettes) who don't know which end of the needle to use.

Designs and Techniques

There is a range of different designs that you could use in a pinch to make a disposable medical face mask. Which design you choose will depend on the materials that you have on hand and the reason for wearing the mask. Each design has pros and cons, so choose carefully.

Basic Design One: The Handkerchief Mask

This is a very easy mask to make, and you could finish it inside of a minute. The speed is its greatest asset, and this makes the handkerchief mask a real asset if you should find yourself exposed to pollutants such as smoke from a burning building, etc.

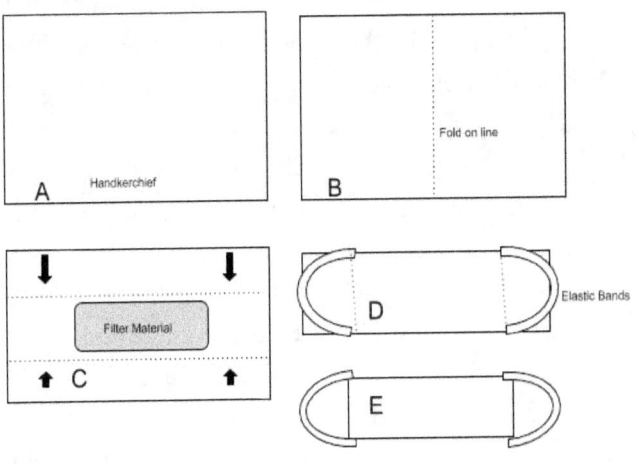

Template four: Handkerchief Mask (Renwick, 2020)

What you'll need:

- One large handkerchief or a square scarf
- Two elastic bands or hair ties

- One square (1.5 x 3 inches) filter material (either cut from a coffee filter or folded kitchen towel)

How to make it:

1. Wash hands or sterilize with hand sanitizer before beginning to make the mask.
2. Fold the handkerchief (A) in half (B), then place and center the filter material (C). Fold the top layers over as in step C.
3. Slip the elastic bands or hair ties over the mask (D), then fold the ends over as in step E.
4. Slip the mask over the face, being careful not to touch the middle part too much. The folded sides should be on the inside of the mask.
5. If you are in a smoky environment, you may soak the filter paper to increase the protection factor. However, if you are protecting against germs, this should be avoided.

Basic Design Two: The Paper Mask

This design is a two-part mask with an optional splatter shield that you could add in extreme cases or if you have to go out in the rain and don't want your mask to get wet. The splatter shield is a regular file pocket that you clip onto your glasses or sunglasses. It hangs loosely over the face and the underlying paper mask, offering 100% protection against liquids that may splash against your face or the paper mask. Though it isn't the most attractive design, it has been found by the Honk Kong Consumer Council to be highly effective.

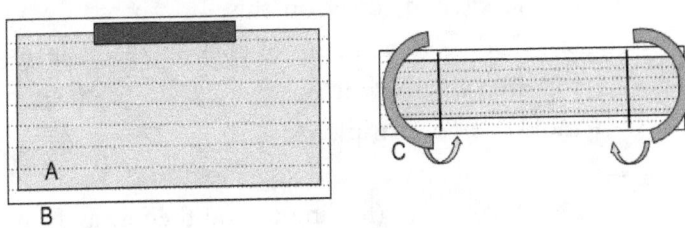

Template Five: Paper Mask (Consumer.org, 2020).

What you'll need:

- Two squares of kitchen paper towels
- Two sheets of tissue paper
- A double-folded strip 1 x 2 inches of aluminum foil (optional)
- Two elastic bands or hair ties

How to make it:

1. Wash and sanitize your hands.
2. Place the first square of the kitchen towel on a firm surface.
3. Place the two sheets of tissue paper on this square.
4. Place the second square of the kitchen towel on this. If you wish, you could add a folded strip of aluminum foil at the top area where your nose would go to create a moldable nose strip (A and B).
5. Now fold the stack of paper like a fan (folding to you then away from you until the zig-zag shape is achieved).
6. Insert the elastic bands or hair ties as in C.
7. Fold the sides of the mask in, flatten slightly, then fit the mask by slipping the elastic bands over your ears.
8. Using the index fingers, gently mold the aluminum strip to fit your nose, creating an effectively sealed edge.
9. Fit the glasses with the splatter shield over this to add a moisture barrier.

This mask design has been proven by the Hong Kong Consumer Council (HKCC) to be 90% as effective as the protection offered by a commercially bought surgical face mask. Additionally, you could try variations of the design. Polypropylene, the materials of non-plastic reusable grocery bags, is similar to the materials of the commercial surgical masks, and this material also offers some water resistance, making it a good choice for replacing the outer paper towel.

Basic Design Three: The T-Shirt Mask

This last design falls within both the disposable and reusable category of DIY medical face masks. It can be washed, and as a bonus, it does not require any sewing. The filter that is used would need to be disposed of and replaced after every wash though, which could present a hygiene problem. You would need to handle the soiled mask, remove a possibly contaminated filter, and dispose of it in a responsible manner. The larger size of the mask also increases the risk of the mask dispersing any trapped biological particles into the air as you remove it. However, given the comfortable fit, quick design, and good protection, it is still worth considering.

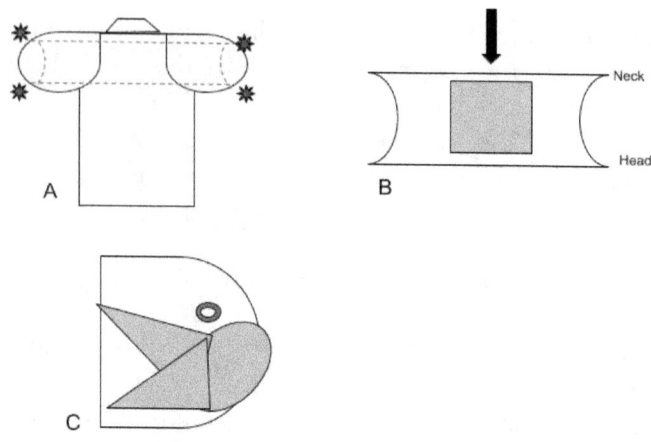

Template Six: T-Shirt Mask (Renwick, 2020).

What you'll need:

- A high-quality T-shirt
- Kitchen towel squares
- Scissors
- A safety pin

How to make it:

1. Wash hands or sanitize appropriately.
2. Using the above template, cut on the red lines, being careful not to cut right through at the four edges of the sleeves marked with a blue star on the design (A).

3. Insert a double-folded paper towel square (3 x 3 inches) into the cut-out (B). Secure the filter part with a safety pin.
4. Place the T-shirt over the face, tying the straps at the bottom of the shape to the head and the top straps to the neck (C).

Whichever mask design you choose, you will need to be responsible to ensure that the disposable masks still offer protection by ensuring a good fit and hygienic disposal of used masks.

Caring for Disposable Masks

Most of the care for disposable medical face masks will be concerned with the safe disposal of these masks. Given that they are mostly made from paper, they are biodegradable. When removing these masks, they should still be placed in a packet of some kind to ensure that they are sealed away to avoid any possible contamination. The safest way to dispose of them is to burn them; however, this may not always be possible. If you are relying on your local refuse services, you should ensure that masks are kept in a sealed packet and labeled as used masks. This should prevent any uninformed persons from trying to wear the masks again.

You could also start the disintegration process by pouring some bleach or rubbing alcohol onto the masks before bagging them. Just because the mask took you a minute to make does not mean that you can simply toss them aside once they have been used. Wearing a medical mask is a responsibility that extends from protecting you to protecting those around you and the environment.

Should your disposable medical face mask have components that may be reused, such as the T-shirt mask, then you need to carefully remove and dispose of the disposable elements such as filters, secure the remaining parts safely, and then wash those in warm water with soap. Dry these parts of the mask in direct sunlight if possible. Do not reuse, wash, or recycle filters.

The temptation may also be there to reuse parts of the mask, such as the elastic bands or nose shaping wires; however, these should be disposed of carefully and never reused. Plastic face shields made from filing pockets may be reused after they have been appropriately sanitized. This can be done by wiping the plastic down with rubbing alcohol and even washing in warm water with soap.

Don't leave the disposal process of your masks to chance. Be prepared and be responsible. You would not leave bullets lying around since those are dangerous. Likewise, you should never leave any form of PPE lying around once it has been used. This includes disposable gloves, disposable and reusable medical face masks, and other medical equipment and clothing.

Rules of Safety for Disposable Masks

Whether your medical face mask is disposable or reusable, there are specific rules to keep you safe while wearing it, during the fitting and removing process, and during the disposal process. Medical face masks are not a substitute for good hygiene practice, and you should wash your hands regularly. This has been said before, but it is repeated due to the great importance of this in avoiding contracting a respiratory infection of any kind.

Safety rules for disposable medical masks include:

1. Before you make your masks, wash your hands thoroughly.
2. Once your mask is completed, fit it immediately or store it in a sealed container such as a Ziplock bag to ensure that it remains uncontaminated for future use.
3. Fit the mask by pulling it straight up to your mouth and nose area. Never slide it over your head or slip it down to your neck.
4. Avoid touching the inside of the medical face mask.
5. Test the edges of the mask to ensure that the mask has created a good fit over your cheeks, chin, and under your eyes.
6. Shape the nose section by pressing on the metal strips or pinching the tissue papers into shape.

7. Ensure that any filters that are fiber-rich are completely covered by secondary layers of tissue to avoid accidentally inhaling any fibers.
8. Once the mask becomes soggy or loses its shape, you should replace it with a fresh mask.
9. Dispose of all used masks responsibly by placing them in a packet, burning, or dissolving them in alcohol.
10. After removing the used disposable mask, wash your hands carefully. Avoid shaking or crumpling the mask as this may disperse contaminants into the air, increasing your risk of harmful exposure.
11. If possible, wash your face as well before fitting a new mask. Check the new mask's fit again. Never assume that a mask is fitting correctly. Check it in the mirror, or use your fingers to check the snugness of your mask's edges.
12. Always keep a fresh mask handy for use. Not having a replacement mask will lead to you no longer being protected if your mask becomes damaged from prolonged wear.

Conclusion

Congratulations! You are now ready to mask up. Having learned all about masks, you will be able to select the best mask to make for you and your family to wear, thereby increasing your protection against airborne diseases and contaminants. In this book, you discovered everything that you needed to know about masks.

Now You Know

Chapter 1 discussed the history of medical face masks, explained why you should be wearing them and the different types of medical face masks and respirators that you may have seen being used in public. This helped you understand the importance of correct fit, safe materials, sanitation practices, and the process of fitting and removing the medical face mask. You also learned the arguments for and against wearing a medical face mask so that you can now make an informed decision about mask use.

Chapter 2 helped you explore the world of reusable medical face masks. You learned all about the reasons to make your own mask, how to care for it, and what materials to choose for making it, and you discovered three exciting patterns for making your own PPE medical face mask. These patterns will encourage you to explore different fits to allow you to decide which design will be more comfortable while still offering optimal protection. From the homemade surgical mask to the basic shaped mask and the duckbill mask, you now have a range of masks at your fingertips. These masks require different levels of sewing abilities, though all three are well within the ability range of even a novice at sewing. This chapter also helped you understand how to store your homemade medical face masks for future use and cleaning purposes. Lastly, you discovered how to choose and use filters that can be inserted into these masks for additional protection.

In Chapter 3, you were offered an alternative to sewn masks with homemade disposable medical face masks. The chapter discussed when and why you might need a disposable face mask, which materials you could use to make one, and how to safely dispose of the mask once it has been worn. The design section explained three very easy designs to follow when making a disposable medical face mask. The handkerchief mask, paper mask, and T-shirt mask all offered moderate protection should you require a disposable mask. The greatest plus of these masks was that they required no sewing skills and could be made in a matter of minutes. Again, you were informed of how to use filters to improve the protection factor of these masks as well as how to correctly fit these to ensure that you received optimum protection. This chapter concluded by explaining why you should follow certain protocols in disposing of these masks as well as explaining how to do so safely.

You now have a wealth of knowledge at your disposal to allow you to make the best possible choice as to which mask to make and wear.

Which Mask Is Right for You?

Wearing a mask is not an alternative to washing your hands or keeping a safe social distance; however, it will increase your chances of avoiding nasty airborne diseases and environmental pollutants that can compromise your respiratory system. By continuously using an effective hygiene practice of wearing masks when you are out in public, in air-conditioned buildings, and if out socially; washing your hands regularly and thoroughly with soap and water; and sanitizing when you are unable to wash your hands, you will be able to avoid diseases and respiratory conditions that can severely affect the quality of your life.

If you are a parent, these practices are part of the life skills that you should teach your children from a young age. The saying goes that when you know better, you do better. Now that you are informed, there is no excuse for laxness and indifference. Be responsible and wear a mask. Here is a recap of some of the considerations that you looked at when choosing a mask:

Any mask you choose needs to be comfortable enough to be worn for extended periods of time. Since you should never slip a mask on and off, it needs to be soft enough on the face to encourage you to wear it continuously or until you need to replace it.

The mask that you choose to make needs to fit correctly. Even an N95 mask will offer limited protection when it is not fitted correctly. Check the area under your eyes and across your nose for a secure fit. Ensure that there are no parts of the mask that suck in air. Elastics and ties should be strong enough to keep the mask in place without you needing to constantly adjust a slipping mask.

Choose materials that offer you comfort and protection. Filters ensure that you can have a flexible mask while still enjoying protection in the filter section. Avoid scratchy materials that will make you fiddle with the mask, and you should never use materials that could be harmful such as using filters containing fiberglass fibers. Before you decide on a new material to use in your homemade medical face masks, you should research the protection factor of that material. A simple Google search will bring a wealth of knowledge to your fingertips. Just because someone is using a certain material in their Pinterest masks does not mean that it is safe or offers good protection.

Lastly, you should consider the quality of airflow that your mask design offers. If you can't breathe normally, you will feel uncomfortable and will likely remove your mask. A lack of sufficient oxygen from breathing incorrectly will also have a severe and negative effect on your body.

Knowledge is power, and you are now empowered to make the best possible decision regarding your and your family's respiratory health. Making and wearing medical face masks can be fun. You can and should involve your children in the making and decorating process. By painting a fun design on your reusable masks, you can mark which mask belongs to which person in the family. Given the global increase in populations and the resulting pollution that industrialization brings, it seems a reality that we will be wearing medical face masks well into the future. By making it a routine, you will ensure that you and your family are prepared and protected.

Finally, you should share knowledge, and we would love it if you could share a review of this book if you found it helpful in teaching you all about making, wearing, and caring for medical face masks.

References

Hamrick, D. (2020). The Coronavirus on Amazon: 44M Medical Masks & 20K Hazmat Suits Sold, Plus Counterfeit Products & More. *https://www.junglescout.com/blog/coronavirus/*

Holmes, C. (n.d.). Face Mask Duckbill With Filter. *https://www.instructables.com/id/Face-Mask-Duckbill-With-Filter/*

Hong Kong Consumer Council. (2020). DIY Face Mask – 8 Steps in Making Protective Gear. *https://www.consumer.org.hk/ws_en/news/specials/2020/mask-diy-tips.html*

Jenkins, J.B. (2020). Homemade Cloth Face Masks: When They Help & How to Keep Them Sterile. *https://healthcare.utah.edu/healthfeed/postings/2020/04/face-masks.php*

Leiva, C. (2020). The Best Materials For DIY Face Masks And Filters.

https://www.huffpost.com/entry/best-materials-diy-face-masks-filters_l_5e8ce4c6c5b6e1a2e0fb4ada?guccounter=1&guce_referrer=aHR0cHM6Ly93d3cuZ29vZ2xlLmNvLnphLw&guce_referrer_sig=AQAAAE4dXnqASGkoYeXgsZ7_t9CjSKv4B5uD6sOC-dJeVMgg8KAtTpanNzz1stUNpuhsz8qv5iywUqMfGvsjuPns-MyvrpAoVyY-y60d9Hk2Ug0Pvc20M1-sRFwveTmbnZ8Uec4p-GZd_6qcs_r3_FDp1-d7kYRijyqeBSjTmet9kZZ1

Novaccivahealth.com. (2019). The History of Disposable Face Masks.

https://www.novaccivahealth.com/2019/08/21/the-history-of-disposable-face-masks/

Renwick, D. (2020). How to Make a Non-Medical Coronavirus Face Mask – No Sewing

Required. *https://www.theguardian.com/us-news/2020/apr/06/how-to-make-no-sew-face-mask-coronavirus*

Robertson, P. (2020). What Are The Best Materials for Making DIY Masks?

https://smartairfilters.com/en/blog/best-materials-make-diy-face-mask-virus/

Waters, M. (2020). A Brief History of Beards and Pandemics.

https://www.vox.com/the-goods/2020/3/30/21195447/beard-pandemic-coronavirus-masks-1918-spanish-flu-tuberculosis

Williams, M. (2020). How to Make Your Own Face Mask at Home.

https://spectrumlocalnews.com/nys/central-ny/news/2020/03/28/how-to-make-your-own-face-mask-at-home